The Little
Book of
Sleep

The Little Book of Sleep

The Art of Natural Sleep

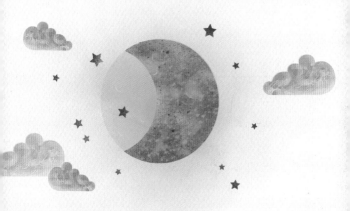

Dr Nerina Ramlakhan

An Hachette UK Company
www.hachette.co.uk

First published in Great Britain in 2018 by Gaia Books,
a division of Octopus Publishing Group Ltd,
Carmelite House, 50 Victoria Embankment,
London EC4Y 0DZ
www.octopusbooks.co.uk

Distributed in the US by Hachette Book Group USA,
1290 Avenue of the Americas, 4th and 5th Floors,
New York, NY 10104

Distributed in Canada by Canadian Manda Group,
664 Annette Street, Toronto, Ontario, Canada M6S 2C8

ISBN 978-1-85675-383-8

A CIP catalogue record for this book is available from the British Library.

Printed and bound in China.

10 9 8 7 6 5 4

Commissioning Editor Leanne Bryan
Art Director Juliette Norsworthy
Senior Editor Pollyanna Poulter
Copy Editor Clare Churly
Designer Sally Bond
Illustrator Abigail Read
Production Controller Dasha Miller

Contents

Introduction

> "Sleep is the golden chain
> that ties health and our
> bodies together"

Thomas Dekker

There's nothing better than a good night's sleep is there? We wake up feeling refreshed, happy and looking forward to the day ahead.

The history of insomnia probably goes back to the time of our earliest ancestors. They lived in a world that was so unsafe that it might have been dangerous to retire to a cave and simply pass out for seven or eight hours on a mat of leaves. We might have become extinct if they had slept like that! So there are times when we don't sleep because we need to be vigilant and to take care of the business of life; and we are well equipped to deal with poor sleep.

Night after night of poor sleep, however, can take its toll. We're designed to spend a third of our lives sleeping and we really do need our sleep. The pace of modern life is fast, and although technology is meant to make things easier for us, instead we've ended up with more demands on our time and energy: longer to-do lists, less downtime and certainly less rest. Unsurprisingly, the use of sleeping pills has increased dramatically in recent years. More people are suffering from exhaustion, burnout and mental health problems. According to the Institute of Medicine, an estimated 50 to 70 million US adults have issues with insomnia and wakefulness. Now, perhaps more than ever, we need our sleep to rebalance, repair and replenish ourselves from the demands of the day.

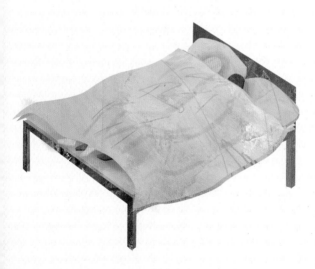

What is a Good Night's Sleep?

What does it mean to get a good night's sleep? It's not just about quantity. It's about getting the right type and quality of sleep.

I use the Sanskrit word *sattvic* to describe the type of sleep we should be getting – pure, deep, natural and healing. This is the kind of sleep where you wake up feeling refreshed, filled with vitality and looking forward to the day ahead. It not only heals us but also heals those around us. We wake up smiling and that energy is contagious; it affects our loved ones, the people we encounter on our journey into work, our colleagues and clients and the very work that we do – the work of life.

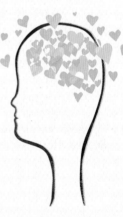

When we sleep deeply, rejuvenation takes place on many levels:

- **Physical:** We wake up with the energy and vitality we need to go about our day's tasks. The body is repaired and the immune system is strengthened.

- **Emotional:** We are able to engage fully in our relationships with courage and open-heartedness and deal with life's inevitable ups and downs.

- **Mental:** The brain is cleaned up and reorganized and we feel creative and focused, even in the face of overflowing inboxes and constant demands from technology.

- **Spiritual:** We can live with meaning, passion and inspiration, finding time for those things that we truly care about.

Sattvic sleep enables us to be the best that we can be – the best version of ourselves and to live our lives with purpose and meaning.

An Innate Ability

Dormancy is part
of the cycle of
life: in order to
thrive, fields must
lie fallow, animals
must sleep or hibernate.
Researchers have been
studying the day and
night cycle in plants
for a long time.

The 18th-century
Swedish naturalist
Carl Linnaeus observed that
flowers in a dark cellar continue to
open and close, and in the 19th century
Charles Darwin recorded the overnight
movement of plant leaves and stalks and
called it "sleep". More recently, scientists
in Austria, Finland and Hungary have
used sophisticated infrared laser scanning
techniques to take pictures of trees
sleeping. Their results (documented

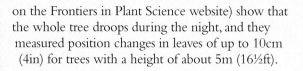

on the Frontiers in Plant Science website) show that the whole tree droops during the night, and they measured position changes in leaves of up to 10cm (4in) for trees with a height of about 5m (16½ft).

A natural process of oscillation is encoded in our DNA. This is well-documented in a field of biology called chronobiology, which is the study of the effect of time – and in particular, rhythms – on living systems. All of nature follows a natural rhythm of energy expenditure and rest.

Sleep is an innate ability that follows an in-built rhythm that is in sync with nature – the periods of light and dark, the changing of the seasons, the waxing and waning of the moon, and the movement of tides. But today's hectic way of life and the constant flood of information bombarding our brain have dulled our connection with this natural ability. In order to get *sattvic* sleep we need to reawaken this knowledge.

If your sleep problems have been going on for a long time, you might feel that it is simply not possible for you to get this type of sleep. I want to reassure you – it is possible. You just need to know how to trigger it.

Live Deeply, Sleep Deeply

If all of nature sleeps, why is it so difficult for us?
Why have we become so disconnected from ourselves?

Electronic devices are amazing, easy to use and so
seductive, but they can have a negative impact on
our health, sleep patterns, energy levels, and even
on our relationships. The problem, however, lies not
with technology, but the way that we're using it. We
constantly live on the surface of life, and in the process
we have lost touch with what lies within us, the true
source of our healing rhythms and bodily wisdom.

To sleep deeply we need to live deeply. This means
that we need to reconnect with ourselves and our
inner stillness. It's not surprising that in the Western
world practices such as yoga and mindfulness have
become popular as more people seek inner peace and
grounding to counterbalance the frenetic pace of life.

Recent scientific studies have shown that spending
time in nature can improve our sleep drastically
by reconnecting us with our innate sleep rhythms.
Kenneth Wright, a researcher at the University of
Colorado Boulder in the USA conducted a study in
2013 (*Entrainment of the Human Circadian Clock to the
Natural Light-Dark Cycle*) in which he sent people

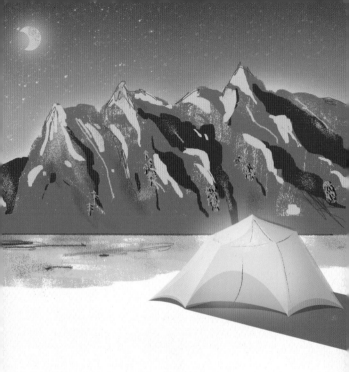

on a week-long summer camping trip to understand
how their internal clocks changed without electronics
and only natural light. Before and after the trip, he
measured their levels of the sleep hormone melatonin.
Wright found that people's internal clocks were
delayed by two hours in their modern environment
but they were able to recalibrate after a week in nature.

A Personal Mission

I'm passionate about helping people to sleep. I have had problems sleeping myself. When I was six months old, in desperation, my mother took me from one doctor to the next to find help. I was such a restless baby. This restlessness continued into my thirties and I became very ill. At this point, I already had a doctorate in neurophysiology but becoming ill set me on a personal mission to learn even more about sleep.

I started going into large companies to give presentations on sleep. For more than a decade I worked in a psychiatric clinic where patients with severe mental health problems needed deep healing sleep. I also worked with Premiership footballers, school children, stressed-out mothers and pop stars. In short, I spent almost 25 years solving all sorts of sleep problems. But I still wanted to learn more…and so I began to delve into ancient Eastern sciences such as Traditional Chinese Medicine and Ayurveda (see pages 22–27).

By merging what I learned from Western science with these older systems of medicine, I began to build a more holistic view of how to help others – and myself – sleep deeply and restoratively.

Sleep is an act of relinquishing control. It's an act of trust and faith. Deep sleep happens when we feel safe. As the Baptist minister Lynn Casteel Harper says, "Learning to honour the body's needs as a sacred part of our design constitutes soul work". So my work with those of you who can't sleep, along with my work on myself, is deep soul work.

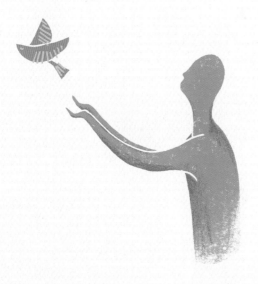

1 The Mystery of Sleep

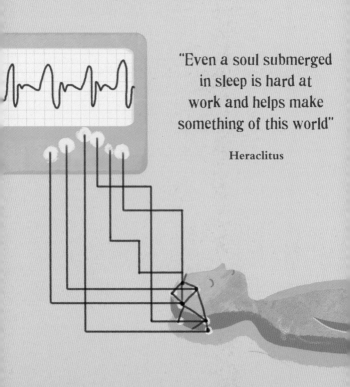

"Even a soul submerged in sleep is hard at work and helps make something of this world"

Heraclitus

Measuring Sleep

Why do we sleep? And what really happens when we sleep? Sleep scientists have been seeking the answers to these questions for a long time. Sleep measurement is usually done in a sleep laboratory. Technicians attach electrodes to the head to take three types of measurement called polysomnography:

- Electrical activity in the brain is measured by electroencephalography (EEG). This measures the different stages of sleep.

- Muscle activity is measured using electromyography (EMG). Muscle tone differs between wakefulness and sleep depending on the stage of sleep.

- Eye movements during sleep are measured using electrooculography (EOG). This helps to identify rapid eye movement (REM) sleep, during which we often dream. The eyeballs make characteristic movements that show us when someone is in this type of sleep.

Sleep Cycles

We sleep in cycles of roughly 90 minutes, called the ultradian cycle. In fact, our energy fluctuates throughout the day in the ultradian cycle so there are times when we feel energized and alert and other times when we just want to have a siesta. Each 90-minute sleep cycle consists of five phases: phases one and two are light sleep, phases three and four are deep sleep and phase five is a 10–15 minute burst of REM sleep.

During sleep our muscles go rigid in order to stop us acting out our dreams. Why do we dream? One theory is that we dream to consolidate the information of the

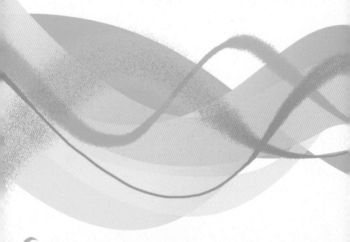

day so that we can wake up feeling mentally focused and alert. During the day our brains are bombarded with information so this process of filing, sifting and sorting is vital to optimize our cognitive function.

As Night Draws In ...

When the sun goes down and the light level in our environment drops below 200 lux, a signal is sent to the pineal gland in the brain to switch on the production of melatonin, which makes us start to feel sleepy. The control centre in the pineal gland is called the circadian timer. The intricate functioning of every cell in the body is regulated by the circadian timer, which is why we experience jet lag when we cross time zones (more on this on page 92).

Your body craves sleep. This is called the sleep drive. Throughout the day, your desire for sleep builds, and when it reaches a certain point you need to sleep. When you're exhausted, your body is even able to engage in microsleep episodes of one or two seconds while your eyes are open. However, napping for too long late in the day can throw off your night's sleep by decreasing your body's sleep drive.

Sleeping Like Our Ancestors

Another perspective on how we sleep comes from studying the sleep patterns of our ancestors. Scientists have examined historical documents that indicate that preindustrial households slept in two cycles, sometimes called "first sleep" and "second sleep".

Each cycle lasted approximately four hours, but there would be two to three hours between the two cycles in which our ancestors could engage in a variety of activities such as talking, reading, praying or physical intimacy. In addition, they might also have had a nap in the afternoon to mop up any fatigue.

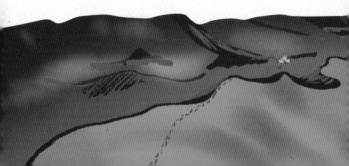

This type of sleeping pattern is called "segmented sleep". It explains why we often wake in the early hours – usually 2am or 3am – feeling quite wide awake. This is normal. In fact, many prolific creative people have been known to do their best work at this time of the day. In today's world, where sleep and rest have become precious commodities and we're constantly looking for ways to be more productive, segmented sleep has become a thing of the past. Now, many of us worry about waking at this time of night. And it is this very worry that can stop us from getting back to sleep again.

Problems can also often seem overwhelming in the early hours, whereas in the clear light of day they may only be minor. Just knowing this could help to pull you out of the worry cycle when you next find yourself awake very early in the morning.

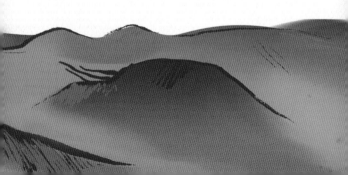

Eastern Perspectives

Western research has advanced our understanding of sleep science but when this knowledge is merged with what ancient cultures have unearthed over thousands of years we can start to create a holistic picture of what sleep really does for us and why it has this tremendous potential to heal.

According to some cultures, deep sleep has a spiritual function that is said to bring about a connection with a Divine source of energy. I've noticed that when people don't sleep well, they become dispirited and begin to lose their *joie de vivre*.

Traditional Chinese Medicine (TCM)

Long ago TCM discovered a "body clock" that can help us understand the way energy moves through our bodies to restore different organ functions. This clock relates to how energy and our organ systems function throughout the whole day. When we look at the night-time portion of the clock (as we have done in the diagram opposite), it gives us a better understanding of why the cycles and phases of sleep are important. It also explains why we need to go to bed and rise at a certain time to stay in optimal health.

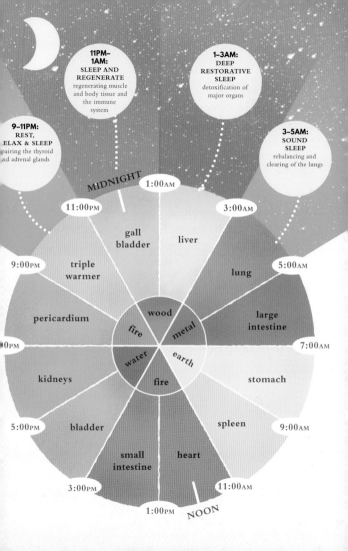

11PM–1AM:
SLEEP AND REGENERATE
regenerating muscle and body tissue and the immune system

1–3AM:
DEEP RESTORATIVE SLEEP
detoxification of major organs

9–11PM:
REST, RELAX & SLEEP
repairing the thyroid and adrenal glands

3–5AM:
SOUND SLEEP
rebalancing and clearing of the lungs

MIDNIGHT

1:00AM

11:00PM

3:00AM

9:00PM

5:00AM

gall bladder

liver

triple warmer

lung

pericardium

large intestine

9:00PM

7:00AM

wood

fire

metal

kidneys

water

earth

stomach

fire

bladder

spleen

5:00PM

9:00AM

small intestine

heart

3:00PM

11:00AM

1:00PM

NOON

Working with so many people over the years has enabled me to build up a picture of what happens emotionally and mentally when we don't sleep well. What I have learned fits with TCM theory and it underlines the importance of getting the right type and amount of sleep and getting into good sleep habits. Repeatedly missing out on vital sleep phases can give rise to both physical and emotional imbalances.

The most important aspects of a good night's sleep are:

- **Winding down in preparation for sleep:** Going to bed or resting between 9pm and 11pm sets us up for good sleep. This vital rest period rebalances the adrenal and thyroid glands and helps to reset and rebalance our metabolism.

- **Levelling out stress hormones:** Also between 9pm and 11pm the sympathetic and parasympathetic nervous system is rebalanced, our adrenaline, noradrenaline and cortisol levels drop off and the feelings of stress you have accumulated during the day level out. The brain also performs a vital cleanup of its filing systems so we can wake up feeling sharp and clear.

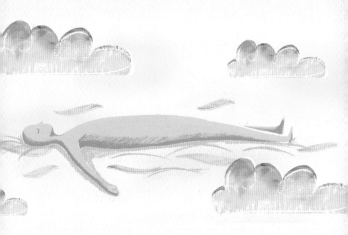

● **Sleeping deeply between 1am and 3am:**
This is the time when deep sleep has the greatest
capacity to heal mind, body and spirit. In TCM
this is called "liver time" because this is when the
liver filters and cleanses the blood and our *qi* (vital
energy or life force) is replenished. Emotions of
fear and anger are also alleviated during this time.

● **Allowing the body time for cleansing:** The
lungs release their waste between 3am and 5am,
which is why this is the time when a smoker
might cough. The emotions of grief and sadness
are soothed during this time.

The Indian Science of Ayurveda

Known as the knowledge of life, Ayurveda can provide us with an insight into sleep and, in particular, sleep imbalances. It is a holistic science that began over 5,000 years ago when Indian monks were looking for different ways to be healthy. They believed that optimizing their health would enable them to develop not just physically but spiritually. They gathered all their conclusions and advice in ancient Sanskrit texts (such as the *Rig Veda*), thus preserving it for future generations.

The Sanskrit word *sattvic* is derived from the word *sattva*, which in Ayurvedic science is one of three *gunas* or qualities of nature or types of energy. The three *gunas* are:

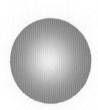

- *Sattva:* Derived from the root word *sat*, meaning "being". This is a state where there is nothing to do, a deeply peaceful and restful stage, the ultimate state of balance.

- *Rajas:* Derived from the root word *raj*, meaning "to glow". This is a state of activity and being on the go, when the mind tends to be overactive.

Tamas: Derived from the root word *tam*, meaning "to perish". In this state of heaviness and dullness, inertia and stagnation, the mind is underactive.

We need a balance of the three *gunas* to think clearly, calmly and creatively and find solutions to life's challenges; the energy of *rajas* enables us to put those solutions into action; and the energy of *tamas* enables us to slow down and bring activities to an end when the challenge has been overcome.

We're aiming for a balanced state of *sattvic* sleep but in this world that is so demanding and *rajassic*, a lot of people find their energy and sleep patterns oscillating wildly between extremes of *rajas* and *tamas*: hyperactive, overstimulated, unable to relax; plummeting to chronic fatigue and illness. The "tired but wired" scenario.

While *sattvic* sleep feels deep and rejuvenating, *rajassic* sleep is fitful, filled with dreams, thoughts, words and even songs with frequent waking and worrying. *Tamassic* sleep is very deep – passing out – with a tendency to oversleep but waking tired, sluggish and wanting more sleep. An imbalance in this *tamas* can even lead to depression and hopelessness.

2 Sleep Issues

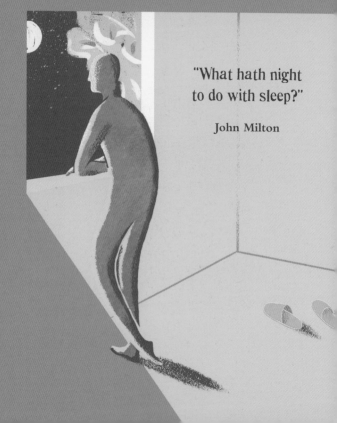

"What hath night
to do with sleep?"

John Milton

Why Can't I Sleep?

The most common sleep problems are:

- Difficulty getting to sleep (sleep initiation).

- Difficulty staying asleep (sleep maintenance).

- Oversleeping and still waking tired (hypersomnia).

- Parasomnias such as nightmares or terrors, sleep walking, sleep talking, grinding teeth (bruxism).

- Restless legs syndrome.

- Snoring and sleep apnoea.

In addition to these, I have identified another type of sleep problem that I call the "Who needs sleep?" disorder. This isn't a recognized disorder but I see so many people who just don't feel they need to sleep. For them sleep is low priority, a luxury, maybe even a weakness. Researchers at the University of Oxford in the UK described this as "sleep arrogance", in which we constantly try to keep up with the demands of life by working against our innate drives and body clock, eking out every last minute to get things done.

You Are Resourceful:
A Case Study

I once worked with a famous athlete – a footballer –
who often worried about not sleeping the night before
a big game. His concern was that he wouldn't be able
to perform at his best the next day if he didn't sleep.

We all experience worries like this from time to
time. It might happen the night before an exam or an
important interview, or the night before your wedding!

A very typical scenario is Sunday Night Syndrome
where you have problems sleeping every Sunday night
in anticipation of the week ahead because you're
telling yourself, "I must sleep well tonight as I've
got a busy week." This problem is sometimes called
the "monkey mind", and this mindset can give rise
to some of the chronic sleep problems I've already
mentioned where the very fear of not sleeping
is what is stopping you from sleeping.

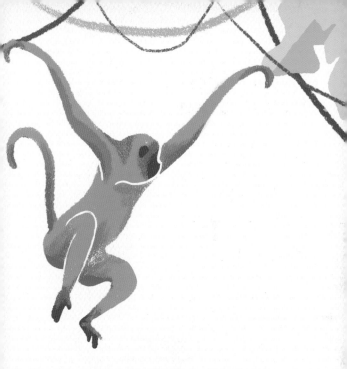

So how do you settle the monkey mind when you need to get to sleep? First of all, you need to stop worrying that a catastrophe will befall you if you don't sleep. Yes, sleep is vital and not sleeping – especially night after night – isn't good for your health and happiness, but you are remarkably well equipped to deal with the odd night of not sleeping well.

Sleep Isn't the Only Way We Get Energy

Our energy doesn't just come from a good night's sleep. It also comes from the food we eat, the exercise we take, the way we breathe, our relationships and the way we think and use our minds. The most important aspect of our energy probably comes from how we nourish our heart and spirit. Think of a time when you fell in love or were excited about a new job or project – you might have found you didn't even need to sleep because you were so excited, and yet you felt fine the next day. In fact, you might have felt energized and happy. And how about those nights when you didn't sleep well before an exam or interview and still managed to do well the next day?

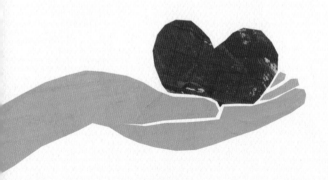

When I explained this to the footballer he started to change his beliefs about sleep. He realized that he'd be fine – even amazing – the next day. As his attitude changed, so did his relationship with sleep. He now sleeps beautifully the night before a big game.

We need to relax our attitude about sleep. Remember, sleep is about relinquishing control. It's about letting go and trusting in our resourcefulness.

Here are some things to reassure you when the monkey mind is stopping you from sleeping:

- It's entirely normal to wake up during the night.

- It's possible to sleep with your eyes open. Yes, you might be getting more sleep than you think (or measure) while you're reading a book or watching TV.

- It's normal not to sleep well sometimes.

So stop worrying. Drop your shoulders, relax the space between your eyebrows, relax your jaw, take a deep breath…then breathe out and let go.

Trust.

And rest.

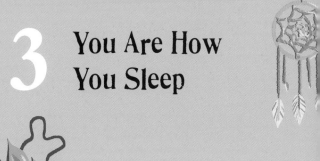

3 You Are How You Sleep

"Early to bed and early to rise, makes a man healthy, wealthy and wise."

Benjamin Franklin

Your Relationship with Sleep

Each of us has a unique relationship with sleep. What is yours?

- What is your relationship with sleep?

- What time do you prefer to go to bed?

- What side of the bed do you prefer to sleep on?

- What do you like to do before you go to bed? And does it really help you to sleep?

- Do you enjoy sleeping?

- Do you view sleep as a priority or is it a luxury – something you do if there's nothing else that needs to be done?

- Do you dread going to bed at night?

- And do you know what you need to do in order to get a good night's sleep?

What Type of Sleeper are You?

One way of looking at your sleeping preference and tendencies is to look at your chronotype – whether you're a morning or an evening person and how this affects your energy rhythms throughout the day. It is thought that your chronotype might be influenced by your genetics, although I believe that our energy and sleep patterns can be significantly influenced by behaviours that we might have learned from childhood and the lifestyle choices we have come to make.

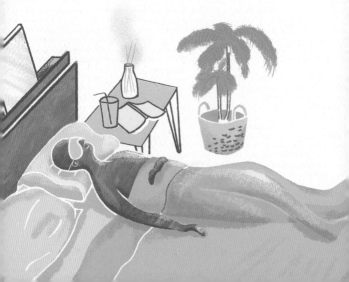

Sensitive Sleepers
and Martini Sleepers

Based on my work with many different types of people over 20 years, I have come up with two categories of sleep types: the Sensitive Sleeper and the Martini Sleeper. My clients have found this distinction helpful because it not only gives them a valuable insight into how they sleep but also into who they are.

If you're a Sensitive Sleeper, you may wake at the slightest sound. You may be sensitive to sights, sounds and smells. What you read or watch on TV and the conversations you have before you go to bed can affect your ability to get to sleep and stay asleep, and can even affect your dreams. Sensitive Sleepers usually prefer to sleep in their own bed and on a certain side of the bed. They tend to have a favourite pillow and may even travel on an airplane with it!

The Sensitive Sleeper can be overly empathetic and in tune with others. Their nervous system can be "skittish" and unsettled, particularly in unfamiliar environments. They feel the sadness and pain of others and can find it hard to let go of the worries of the day. They find it difficult to sleep on a problem and need to feel settled and peaceful in order to sleep restfully.

In contrast, Martini Sleepers may actually sleep on a problem! They can sleep any time, any place, anywhere – the well-known strapline from a 1970s Martini advertisement. Martini sleepers don't understand all the fuss about sleeping. You just do it, don't you? However, they can fall prey to oversleeping (see page 29) or hypersomnia and then wake feeling sluggish and unmotivated.

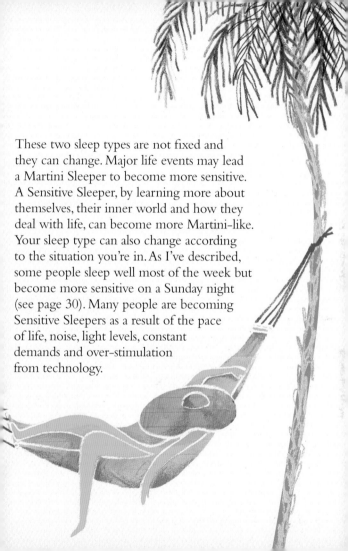

These two sleep types are not fixed and
they can change. Major life events may lead
a Martini Sleeper to become more sensitive.
A Sensitive Sleeper, by learning more about
themselves, their inner world and how they
deal with life, can become more Martini-like.
Your sleep type can also change according
to the situation you're in. As I've described,
some people sleep well most of the week but
become more sensitive on a Sunday night
(see page 30). Many people are becoming
Sensitive Sleepers as a result of the pace
of life, noise, light levels, constant
demands and over-stimulation
from technology.

An Ayurvedic Perspective

Ayurveda (see page 26), like Traditional Chinese Medicine (see page 22), believes that every individual is unique and there is no "one size fits all" solution. According to Ayurveda, every individual is made up of a unique combination of three main *doshas* or energies, which give them their unique physiology and psychology.

The *doshas* are:

Vata: The "air" energy that's related to motion – heartbeat, circulation, breathing, blinking

Pitta: The "fire" energy that's related to metabolic systems including digestion, absorption, nutrition and body temperature

Kapha: The "water" energy that's related to growth in the body. It maintains the water balance in the body, moisturizes the skin and maintains the immune system.

Imbalances of the *doshas* give rise to not only physical ailments but also sleep disturbances.

Vata	Overthinking, unable to fall asleep and/or stay asleep, feeling tired but wired, worrying about the day's events, unable to stop thinking, shallow and restless sleep, waking tired.
Pitta	No problem falling asleep but waking in the early hours and unable to get back to sleep. People who are experiencing stress and emotional trauma are prone to this.
Kapha	Oversleeping or hypersomnia. The person sleeps long and deeply but still feels exhausted on waking. Lethargy and dullness persist throughout the day.

Sleep Right For Your Type

Vata: Avoid mental overstimulation at night. A regular wind-down routine is important. Aim to be in bed early – around 9.30pm – to calm your mind. Work on letting go to calm the *vata* element.

Pitta: Keep your bedroom cool. Sprinkle eucalyptus oil on your pillow. Avoid competitive exercise close to bedtime. Avoid overly spicy foods at night-time and minimize your intake of caffeine and alcohol.

Kapha: Wake up early – ideally before 6am. Set an alarm clock – several if necessary – and put it in another part of the bedroom so you have to get up to switch it off. Vigorous exercise in the morning is good. Keep active during the day and avoid sitting for too long. Eat lightly in the evening and avoid heavy carbohydrate-based meals.

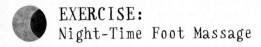

EXERCISE:
Night-Time Foot Massage

Foot massage is said to balance the *doshas* so we can all benefit from doing this – even the watery, Martini-like *kapha* types. The simple act of rubbing oil on the soles of the feet – especially at bedtime – calms *vata* and can really help to quiet the thoughts and slow down a racing mind.

1 Create a lovely ambience for your foot massage: light a candle or play some relaxing music.

2 Warm a small amount of massage oil – preferably coconut oil – and begin to slowly massage the soles of your feet using circular movements with your thumb. Continue doing this for 10 minutes or until all of the oil has been absorbed into the skin. Take your time and enjoy the sensation of caring for one of the most neglected areas of your body. Think loving thoughts as you do this massage – let it be a meditation.

3 When you are finished, put on some warm cotton socks, get into bed and prepare to sleep like a baby.

4 From Surviving to Thriving

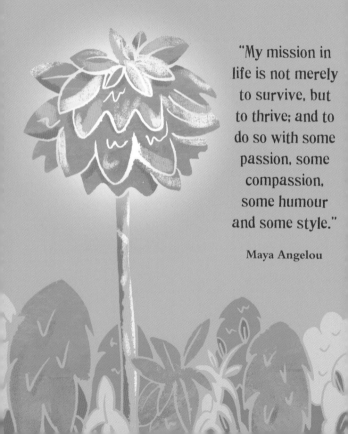

"My mission in
life is not merely
to survive, but
to thrive; and to
do so with some
passion, some
compassion,
some humour
and some style."

Maya Angelou

When Your Nervous System is Nervous

How did you feel when you woke up this morning? Did you wake with a smile on your face, looking forward to the day ahead? Or was your mind racing, thinking of all the have-to-dos, should-dos, must-dos?

Did you pick up your phone and dive into your inbox as soon as you woke? Was your stomach in a knot? Did you skip breakfast but reach for a cup of tea or coffee? The world is going so fast that many people are living in survival mode, constantly living in the future, unable to savour and enjoy the present moment.

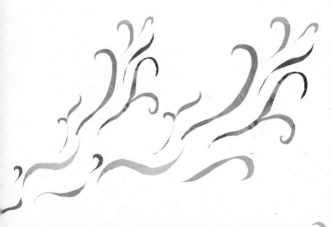

Understanding your Nervous System

Our nervous system is intelligently designed for both survival and safety. Depending on what is happening in our external world, it will help us to survive and fight threat if we need to or to thrive and live life joyfully and restfully.

The autonomic nervous system is divided into two branches – the so-called fight or flight or sympathetic nervous system (SNS) and the parasympathetic nervous system (PNS), which allows us rest, repair, heal and sleep. If we feel anxious, fearful and distrusting of life, we will tend to live in our SNS. But if we feel safe, peaceful and happy then we are living in our PNS … and we will sleep deeply and restoratively.

In other words, it is impossible to sleep well if we are running in survival mode. This is a physiological adaptation that we've had since the days of living in the wilderness as hunter-gatherers but it may not be that helpful in today's world.

Feel Safe, Sleep Deeply

When we feel safe – in our mind, our body, our nervous system – we will experience *sattvic sleep*. But what does it mean to feel safe? It means that deep within we feel steady and stable regardless of what's going on in our lives. It's so easy to feel that our world simply isn't safe and, if we constantly bombard our minds with information that reinforces this belief, it's no wonder that we can't sleep at night.

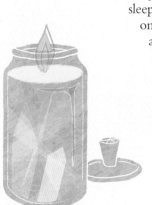

So the journey back to deep sleep is about working on yourself to create an inner core of safety, and making lifestyle choices that will help your nervous system to recalibrate and shift back into safety mode if you've been running in survival mode.

Steps Toward Feeling Safe

The first step toward feeling safe is to work with your breath. On average we breathe 20,000–25,000 times a day, and most of our breathing is unconsciously driven. Often, if we're living in survival mode, our breathing is shallow and inefficient. We might actually be breathing in a way that makes us feel more stressed and adrenalized, causing tightness in our neck and shoulders, which leads to headaches and sleeplessness.

The way we breathe also affects whether the SNS or PNS is active. If you're anxious and breathing in a rapid and shallow way from your chest, your SNS will be predominantly active. If you are relaxed and breathing slowly and deeply from your belly, you will be activating the vagus nerve that runs through the diaphragm and activates the PNS.

In other words, you can literally breathe your way into a state of survival or safety. If you want to change your relationship with sleep, you need to start by taking some baby steps. Becoming aware is the first step to taking responsibility…and when we take responsibility we might make different choices.

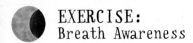

EXERCISE:
Breath Awareness

1 Put this book down and become aware of your
   breathing. Have you been holding your breath
   while reading or did reading about breathing
   make you focus on your breath?

2 Place your left hand on your chest just over your
   heart and your right hand just above your belly
   button. Notice how your hands
   move as you breathe. Just
   notice. That's all you have
   to do. Don't try to change
   your breathing. Let it do
   whatever it wants to
   do. Simply become
   aware of it.

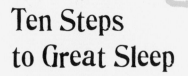

5 Ten Steps to Great Sleep

"A journey of a thousand miles begins with a single step."

Lao Tzu

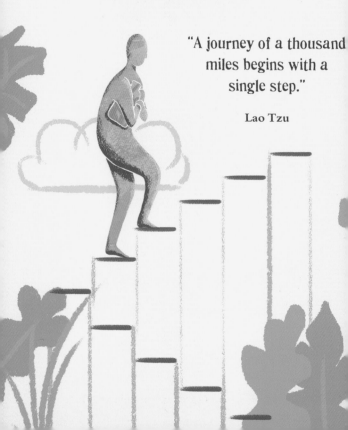

Tried-and-tested Tips

I'm going to share ten tips that will make a big difference to how you sleep. I learned these things by trying and testing them not only on the thousands of people I've worked with but also on myself – and they work. Start doing these things today – even if you're on sleeping tablets (don't come off them suddenly), and they will start to make a difference in 7 to 10 days. Ideally, stick with them for 21 to 28 days to create lifetime habits.

1 Eat within 30 minutes of rising.

2 Reduce your caffeine intake.

3 Drink plenty of water.

4 Get an early night.

5 Stop measuring!

6 Take breaks from technology.

7 Create a sanctuary in your bedroom.

8 Get physical.

9 Let go.

10 Connect with nature.

Eat Within 30 Minutes of Rising

1

Breakfast is particularly important if you wake up and your nervous system is in survival mode. Even a modest breakfast, such as eight almonds and two dates, can be enough to kick-start your metabolism and stabilize your blood sugar levels. Eating within 30 minutes of rising stops your body moving into survival mode and switches it into "safety" mode.

Over time your metabolism will respond and you will start to wake up feeling hungrier. Then you can slowly increase the size of your breakfast and become more creative with your breakfast options. To start with, try:

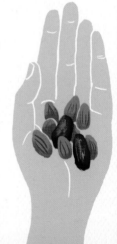

- A small smoothie made with oats, coconut or almond milk, chia seeds, fruit, protein powder or ground almonds.

- A piece of toast with nut butter.

- A small handful of nuts and a piece of fruit.

- A boiled egg.

2 Reduce Your Caffeine Intake

Caffeine mimics the effect of adrenaline. It keeps you wired and stuck in survival mode, which switches off the PNS (see page 46) and sleep system.

Aim to consume less than 300mg of caffeine per day or none at all if you're really struggling to sleep. As a guide, one cup of instant coffee contains around 80mg of caffeine.

The half-life of caffeine (the time taken for the level of caffeine in your blood to drop by 50 percent) is 5 hours. This means if you have a cup of coffee or tea at 5pm, you'll still have half the amount of caffeine in your system at 10pm, so it's best to avoid it after 3pm.

Many people who are stuck in survival mode find it hard to eat and need to drink caffeine to get going. You can break this fatigue cycle by eating a small breakfast (see opposite for some suggestions) and avoiding any caffeine until you've eaten.

3 Drink Plenty of Water

The human body is made up of 70–80% water, and we need to be well hydrated in order for our sleep biochemistry to function optimally. Dehydration can wake you during the night and can actually worsen night sweats. Ideally, you should drink 1.5–2 litres (2½–3½ pints) of water per day – this includes herbal teas, diluted squash and fruit juice but not alcohol or caffeinated drinks, which are diuretics (these make you lose more fluid than you actually retain). Get into the habit of keeping a bottle of water with you at all times and sip from it throughout the day. Try adding fresh herbs, ginger or fruit to enhance the taste.

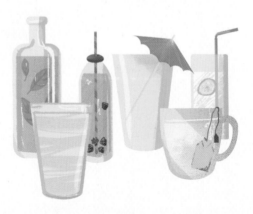

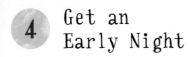

4 Get an Early Night

It's important to allow ourselves time to rest and restore our energies. Remember, according to Traditional Chinese Medicine (see page 22), the few hours before midnight is the best time to erase the stress of the day, reduce adrenaline levels, rebalance the immune system and prepare the body for *sattvic* sleep.

Start preparing to rest and wind down between 9pm and 9.30pm. You don't have to be in bed and fast asleep, but avoid technology, over-stimulation and watching the news. Instead, read something relaxing and uplifting. If possible, avoid stressful conversations.

The aim is to enter a "safety zone", to feel peaceful, calm and in a receptive state to receive deep sleep.

If you can do this four nights per week you will really start to notice a difference in your health and energy levels.

5 Stop Measuring!

It's completely normal to wake during the night. What isn't normal or helpful is to obsess about the time you wake up or calculate how much sleep you may or may not get. To help you do this, turn your clock to face away from the bed and try not to check the time when you wake during the night.

If you are using a device or app to monitor your sleep, bear in mind that this may make you feel more anxious and worried and such tools are not entirely accurate. As a simple guideline, if measuring your sleep is making you worry, stop doing it.

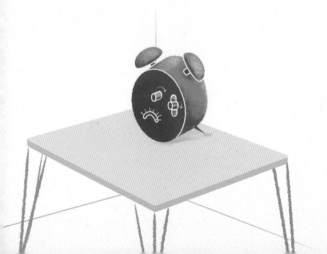

6 Take Breaks From Technology

Create an electronic sundown and withdraw from technology an hour before you get into bed. Don't keep your phone in your bedroom or watch TV in bed. If you wake up during the night (remember – this is normal, see page 21), don't check your phone and definitely don't look at emails.

Taking breaks from technology during the day – ideally a few minutes every 90 minutes or so – is also important. It allows your nervous system moments to settle and be still and enables the brain to engage in vital mental processing, which will help you to sleep more deeply at night because there's less filing work for the brain to do.

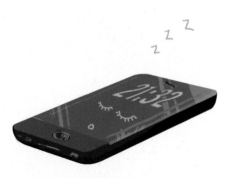

7 Create a Sanctuary in Your Bedroom

Stand in your bedroom, take a deep breath and allow yourself to absorb the feel of the room. Ask yourself: How does it feel? How does it smell? Is it tidy or messy, cosy or impersonal? Do you love your bed? Is your mattress uncomfortable? Does your bedroom make you feel peaceful and mellow? Does it help you to let go of the day? Does it make you feel safe or does it make you feel restless, anxious and tense?

Your bedroom should be an oasis of calm and tranquillity which means paying close attention to sights, sounds and smells. To turn your bedroom into a sanctuary:

- Choose soft, relaxing colours for your bed linen and curtains.

- Consider getting a new mattress if your current one is more than seven years old.

- Place objects that are special to you on your bedside table.

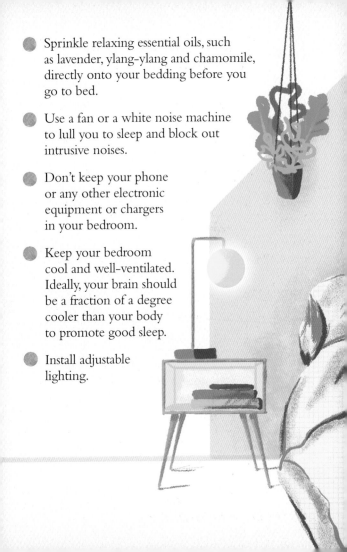

- Sprinkle relaxing essential oils, such as lavender, ylang-ylang and chamomile, directly onto your bedding before you go to bed.

- Use a fan or a white noise machine to lull you to sleep and block out intrusive noises.

- Don't keep your phone or any other electronic equipment or chargers in your bedroom.

- Keep your bedroom cool and well-ventilated. Ideally, your brain should be a fraction of a degree cooler than your body to promote good sleep.

- Install adjustable lighting.

8 Get Physical

Physical movement can help us produce
the chemical adenosine, which promotes
sleepiness and enables melatonin
to work more effectively.

You don't have
to do huge
amounts of
intense activity
– just getting
up and moving
every hour or so
throughout the day
is beneficial.

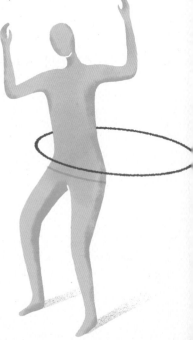

Here are some small ways to incorporate regular movement into your day:

- Stand with your feet hip-width apart. Engage your stomach muscles, stand tall, roll your shoulders down and back and breathe deeply. Stretch your arms wide and up to the sky.

- Sit and lean forward over your knees to stretch out your lower back and shoulders, allowing your arms and hands to dangle like a rag doll.

- Open your mouth as wide as you can in a soundless scream and poke your tongue out at the same time. Open your eyes wide and roll them clockwise and anticlockwise in the sockets.

- To really get things moving, get some juggling balls or a hula hoop. And use them!

The more times you inhabit your body during the day, the easier it will be for you to feel your way into deep sleep at night.

9   Let Go

Sleep will come more effortlessly if you can let go of the day before you get into bed.

There will always be some unfinished business – for example, unresolved conflict with your teenager or worry about your aging parent – but when you put your head on the pillow you need to be able to let go of it all for now and accept restoration.

Here are some ways to help you let go of the day:

● Write a list before you leave work or, at least, before you get into bed. Don't carry it in your head all night because this is what will awaken you in a state of panic and worry at 2am.

● Leave a notebook on your bedside table in case you wake up during the night and remember something that has to be done.

● Write about the problem in a journal to release it from your mind.

● Take some time out to sit and meditate, using this two-step *kshepana mudra* (hand gesture), to point your worries up and away from you:

1 Interlock your fingers, then release your index fingers so they are joined and pointing upward. Place your hands in front of your heart or above your head with your arms straight.

2 Close your eyes or focus on a fixed point ahead of you and hold the mudra for 3–5 minutes while breathing deeply into your belly.

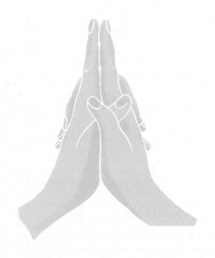

Connect with Nature

Studies show that getting out into nature, ideally somewhere green or near water and trees, helps to restore the balance of the hormones serotonin, oxytocin and melatonin that are vital for your mood, wellbeing and sleep.

To restore your connection with the Earth, try this exercise. It is especially powerful if you do it before you go to bed at night, although you might need to wash your feet afterwards!

1 Stand with bare feet hip-width apart on a patch of damp earth, grass or sand. If the ground is dry, fill a jug or watering can with water and pour water over your feet as you stand there.

2 Soften your knees by bending them slightly and feel the spread of your feet on the ground. Lift your toes and plant them back down.

3 Breathe deeply and as you exhale send that breath down into your belly and out through your feet. Imagine you are breathing roots out from your feet. Use your breath to send those roots deeper and

deeper down into the Earth. Imagine those roots becoming strong and thick. Give them a colour.

4 As you breathe in, imagine drawing healing energy up through those roots and into your body. Imagine this healing energy washing away the fiery energy of the day and any stuck or stale energy lodged in your body. Send that energy out of your body through the roots.

5 If it feels right, add some small movements such as shaking or swaying into the practice while keeping your feet firmly rooted and grounded, or simply stand still and strong. Do this for 3–5 minutes.

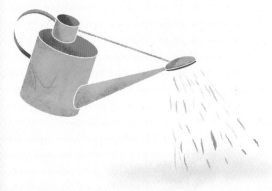

6 Feel Your Way to Sleep

"The body is the shore on the ocean of being."

Anonymous

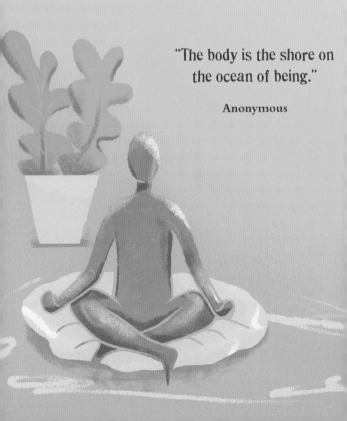

Sleep is a Felt Experience

We spend too much time inside our heads.
So it's unsurprisingly that when we get into
bed we're still thinking about the day we've
had, what we should or shouldn't have said
or done, and what we need to say or do
the following day. We're not present
in our body.

Some people are even
uncomfortable with the sensations
in their body when they get into
bed at night. They drift off, only
to wake up with a jolt as they
begin to fall asleep, which can
feel quite alarming. This is called
a hypnagogic jerk.

So how do we ease ourselves back
into our body in a way that feels safe
and soothing? Start by following the
exercises in this chapter.

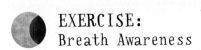

EXERCISE:
Breath Awareness

Do this exercise at least once a day. Ideally, as soon as you wake up, a few times during the day and at night as you're drifting off to sleep. You don't have to sit for 5–10 minutes each time, simply bring your attention to your breathing and notice it. That's all you have to do. Try it if you wake during the night. It's a simple way of taking yourself effortlessly into a state of rest.

1 Sit comfortably on a chair or cross-legged on the floor and close your eyes.

2 Notice whatever you notice – the sounds around you, sensations in your body, thoughts drifting through your mind. Notice your breathing. Just allow it to do whatever it wants to do. Don't try to change it, just allow it to follow its own rhythm and pace.

3 Now label your breaths. As you breathe in, silently and softly whisper "in". As you breathe out, whisper "out". Your inner voice should be soft and sweet, as if you're putting a baby to sleep.

4 Sit like this for 5–10 minutes, just following your breaths with these soft inner whispers.

The more you practise breath awareness, the more it becomes part of your way of being. Eventually you might not even need to be consciously aware of your breathing – it will happen efficiently of its own volition. This is when you will naturally start to experience *sattvic* sleep.

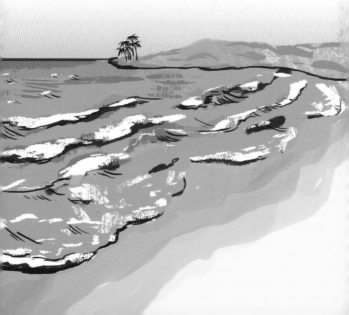

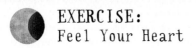

EXERCISE:
Feel Your Heart

One of the most effective ways of coming back into your body after a busy day is to feel the power of your heart, which becomes even stronger when you're feeling grateful.

1   Sit or lie down in a quiet space. Bring to mind an image of someone you love, someone for whom you feel profoundly grateful. It might well be someone you encountered today or someone you haven't seen for a while or even someone who has passed away.

2   Imagine them standing in front of you. Look into their eyes and say, "Thank you, I love you, thank you for being in my life."

3   Breathe into the feeling in your heart as you feel the love and gratitude for them. Imagine a beautiful light growing from the centre of your heart. Give it a colour. See this light growing bigger and brighter until it fills your entire chest area and then your whole body.

4   Send some of this loving light to the person you are thinking about. You might want to expand this light even more and send it to everyone you love. Or you

could send it to those people who you don't love, the ones who cause you unhappiness or stress – they will especially benefit from your loving light.

5 Send your light to the entire world. Imagine it encircling the planet and bringing love and healing to all. Rest in this beautiful light glowing from your heart.

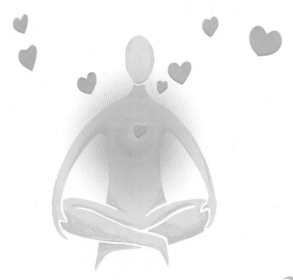

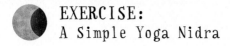

EXERCISE:
A Simple Yoga Nidra

Yoga *nidra* is deeply replenishing and restorative. You can do this exercise mid-afternoon for 10–15 minutes or use the sequence to lull you into deep *sattvic* sleep.

1 Lie back and relax into the floor or bed. Allow yourself to be deeply supported. Become aware of your breathing. Follow the in and out of your breath.

2 Feel inside your heart and find a safe space within it, maybe by thinking of someone you're grateful for or sending love to someone in your life who makes you feel secure and protected.

3 Go even deeper inside and notice your heart's deepest longing. What does your heart truly desire? Create a *sankalpa*, an intention affirmation based on your heart's longing. Word it positively and in the present tense as if it's already happening, for example, "I flow through life with ease and peace. I am relaxed." or "I am safe. All is well in my world."

4 Allow your awareness to travel through your body. Notice any areas of tightness and breathe into that area to relax the tightness. Focus on your face, the space between your eyes, your cheeks, your jaw. Relax your tongue, relax your shoulders, relax and soften your belly.

5 Come back to noticing your breath. Notice the natural in and out rhythm of your breath. As you exhale, imagine a wave passing downward through your body, carrying tensions, fears, worries and anxieties out through your feet. Send them down to the earth. As you inhale, imagine a fresh wave flowing upward through your whole body, bringing a sense of peace, serenity and safety to every tissue, muscle and cell of your body. Surrender to the feeling of deep peace and safety.

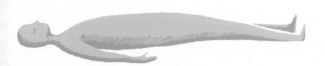

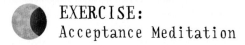

EXERCISE:
Acceptance Meditation

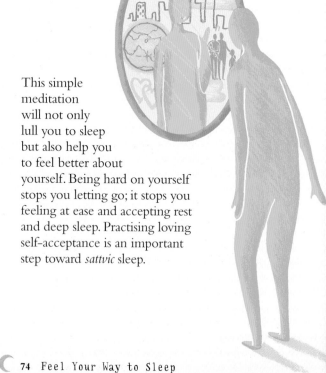

This simple
meditation
will not only
lull you to sleep
but also help you
to feel better about
yourself. Being hard on yourself
stops you letting go; it stops you
feeling at ease and accepting rest
and deep sleep. Practising loving
self-acceptance is an important
step toward *sattvic* sleep.

1 Lie down on your bed and relax. Enjoy the sensation of being supported, the smell and feel of your bed linen.

2 Close your eyes and bring your attention to your breath. Notice the natural rhythm of your breath.

3 Bring your attention to your feet, saying,

"I love my right foot.
I love my toes.
I love my right instep.
I love my right ankle.
I love the top of my right foot.
I love my left foot."

4 Continue to work your way up your body, acknowledging your love for every part of you. Do this very slowly and very gently, as if you're speaking to baby. There's no rush. If you fall asleep and then awaken, start all over again from your feet.

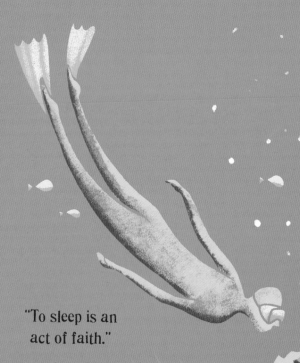

7 Going Deeper

"To sleep is an act of faith."

Barbara Grizzuti
Harrison

Feel Good, Sleep Deeply

When we do the things that we truly care about, such as reading a book, or making time for the people we love, we produce a cocktail of feel-good hormones such as oxytocin and serotonin. These are the hormones that enable us to have faith and trust life. They make us feel safe, and when we feel safe we sleep deeply.

Here are some simple – but powerful – ways to increase your oxytocin levels:

- Express your feelings.

- Have a massage.

- Hug someone.

- Stroke your pet.

- Do something kind for someone.

- Pray.

Focus on What You Care About

It's relatively easy to focus on the things you care about when life is quiet but it's not so easy when life is challenging. However this is the time when you most need to connect with what you care about. It could be as simple as taking 5 minutes to sit and daydream while drinking tea from your favourite mug or putting on your favourite piece of music and dancing to it as if no one's watching.

Try to do something you care about every day – no matter how small. Notice when you feel the urge to mindlessly pick up your phone or surf the internet and instead do something you love.

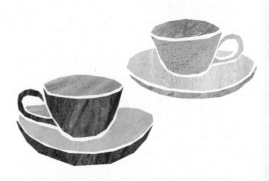

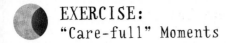

EXERCISE:
"Care-full" Moments

The more "care-full" moments you have in your day, the deeper you will sleep at night. Use this exercise to recognise and consciously embrace these moments.

1 Find a quiet space and light a candle. Have a notebook and pen beside you.

2 Sit quietly, close your eyes and tune in. Think about a time when you felt at your best, happy and carefree. (It need not have been for a long period of time. It might just be a moment.) What were you doing?

3 Go back in your memory and capture as many of these moments as possible. Write them down in your notebook.

4 Make a commitment to bring as many of these small things back into your life as possible. When will you do them? How will you make them non-negotiable? Make a plan.

Dream Journalling

Our dreams can contain insights into what we truly
care about and long for. Keep a journal and pen on
your bedside table and write your dreams down as
soon as you wake in the morning. Do this as a stream
of consciousness. Just write whatever you recall
from your dreams and you'll become more adept
at capturing them and understanding their meaning.
You may not understand them at the time but a chance
happening or conversation later in the day may trigger
an insight that brings you some clarity.

When we begin to follow our dreams, life can change
profoundly, opening up more opportunities, enabling
us to take risks or a leap of faith – but with a deeper
sense of knowing and inner guidance.

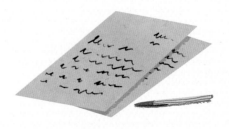

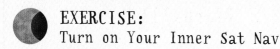

EXERCISE:
Turn on Your Inner Sat Nav

Everyone has an internal guidance system that helps them to make more powerful choices that guide them in the right direction. I call this your inner sat nav. It is made up of your values – those inner traits that are most important to you and which guide your smallest everyday choices.

Set aside some uninterrupted time to reflect on this exercise and keep a notebook and pencil handy to journal your insights.

1 Write down the key words that describe how you want to live your life.

2 Connect with these words regularly, several times a day, for the next 21 days. Notice how they begin to guide your choices.

3 Notice what you start to say yes and no to. Notice what happens to your sleep.

8 Sleep and Life

"I love sleep. My life has a tendency to fall apart when I'm awake, you know?"

Ernest Hemingway

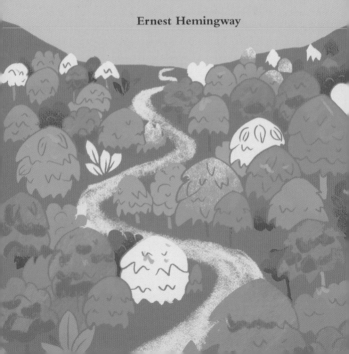

Adapt to Life's Changes

Just like the branches of a tree bending in a storm, there are times when we have to adapt and flex to meet the changing requirements of life. Nothing stays the same – we are constantly growing and renewing – and our relationship with sleep can reflect this too.

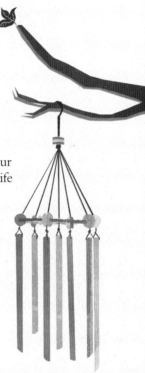

We change as we grow older, as our physiology alters, as our external life circumstances shift. The key is to stay mindful and in touch with ourselves, listening deeply to our body and its differing needs so that we can move with the changes … and continue to sleep peacefully at night.

Sleep During Pregnancy

During pregnancy your physiology changes
and adapts in line with your baby's development.
Hormonal changes, nausea, fatigue, heartburn,
mood changes and anxiety can all affect your sleep,
particularly in the third trimester of pregnancy when
physical discomfort may make you restless. Your sleep
pattern starts to adapt to that of your baby's; you may
wake more frequently and sleep more shallowly. You
may even dream more vivid and surreal dreams.

Ayurvedic medicine stresses that these changes are
essential to the developing baby and the discomfort
can be minimized by maintaining a way of life that's
as pure or *sattvic* as possible. This means maintaining
good sleep habits, getting regular exercise, eating little
and often, avoiding heavy meals, refined sugars and
caffeine and drinking enough fluids.

Paying attention to your baby's rest–activity cycle is
the best guide to know when you should be active
or resting. This is the ideal time to practise napping.
If you can't sleep, put the focus on resting instead.

A pregnant woman is far more able to cope with the
changes to her sleep than a woman who isn't pregnant.
Rising levels of pregnancy hormones, in particular

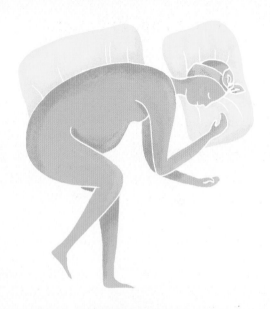

oxytocin, bolster your resilience to all these changes making you more optimistic and trusting of the amazing process your body is going through.

Pregnancy can bring up some classic worries: How will I cope with the birth? Will I bond with my baby? Will I know what to do? We have to remember that we have centuries of amazing mothering capacity built into our DNA. Connect to Mother Earth (see page 88). Breathe in trust. Breathe out fear.

Sleep and Your Child

Children need to feel safe in order to be able to sleep. Their fertile imaginations can make scary monsters of what happens in their day, either stopping them falling asleep or waking them suddenly during the night with nightmares and night terrors. Some children may grind their teeth at night and this can be related to the frustration of not being able to express their feelings.

Some children are naturally good sleepers while others are more sensitive. Most children fall somewhere between these two extremes. It's important to get them into good routines and habits.

It's also important to encourage children to express themselves as much as possible, to talk about what's worrying them or even write about it or draw pictures. The key is to get it out so it doesn't spill into their sleep. Ideally, encourage your child to talk about their worries during the day rather than in bed at night, although you may find this is the time when they will want to talk.

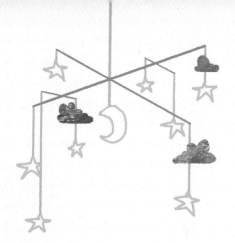

 EXERCISE:
The Perfect Bedtime Story

1 Make your child comfy in bed then ask them
  to think of as many nice things as possible that
  happened in their day.

2 They might need some initial prompting. Help
  them to focus on really little things rather than
  trying to look for big things – for example, the
  sun shining, or something a friend or teacher
  said to them. Try to help them find the silver
  lining in even seemingly negative situations.

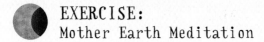

EXERCISE:
Mother Earth Meditation

This is a beautiful exercise for connecting with a deep place of trust within yourself and, if you are pregnant, for strengthening the bond between you and your baby. Particularly useful if you can't sleep at night.

1 Sit or lie using pillows, bolsters or cushions to get really comfy. If you like, light a candle and play your favourite relaxing music.

2 Close your eyes. Connect to the natural rhythm of your breathing.

3 On an out breath, imagine sending roots down to the centre of Mother Earth. Imagine those roots. Give them a colour. Make them strong and thick.

4 Breathe in and imagine drawing in the light of beautiful Mother Earth through those roots – give it whatever colour you choose. Visualize this light entering your body and filling every part of you. See this light enveloping you (or you and your baby). Know that this light holds you in a protective bubble, filling every cell of your body with age-old mothering wisdom.

Sleep and The Menopause

During menopause, women often experience hormonal imbalances that can cause unpleasant symptoms, such as hot flushes and insomnia. This life stage can be navigated with greater ease by paying special attention to self-care and drawing on the support of TCM and Ayurveda.

Herbal remedies and acupuncture can offer gentle support with minimal side effects. Find a TCM practitioner who offers you individualized treatment.

In Ayurveda, menopause is a shift from the *pitta* (fiery, action-based) to the *vata* (slower, gentler) phase of life. Focus on making kinder lifestyle choices, such as allowing yourself to rest, and eating the right foods. Avoid *pitta* foods (such as chillies, caffeine, and alcohol), which exacerbate hormonal imbalances, and cook with calming spices, such as cardamom and fennel.

Pay attention to what your body and mind need. Pamper yourself, use cooling aromatherapy oils, such as peppermint, to avoid overheating at night and plan your power naps! Connect regularly to Mother Earth (see opposite) and remind yourself that your body is wise and has all the intelligence it needs to navigate this phase of life.

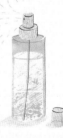

Shared Caves

Sharing your sleep space with another human being is one of the most enjoyable ways of building intimacy but it can also be one of the most frustrating. Many people struggle because they simply can't sleep when lying next to someone – particularly if one of you is a Sensitive Sleeper and the other is a Martini Sleeper (see page 37).

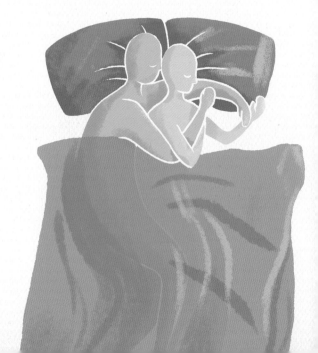

Here are a few things that may help to ease the situation for you and your partner:

- Get the biggest bed you can fit in your bedroom, ideally designed so your partner's movements don't disturb you.

- Change your mattress every seven years or so as it loses its elasticity and supportive properties.

- White noise or at least a fan in the room can act as a buffer against intrusive snores and snuffles.

- Increase your hydration levels and reduce alcohol intake.

- Exercise regularly to tone the respiratory airways and maintain a healthy weight.

- Plan when you will sleep together and when you'll sleep apart, depending on your level of tiredness and what's happening the next day.

Travel and Jet Lag

When you travel by plane, train or car, your body moves faster than nature intended it to. High-speed travel introduces an ungrounded, spaced-out quality into your body and mind. It also disrupts your daily routine and can pull 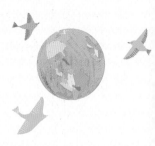 you across time zones. All this aggravates the *vata dosha* (see page 40), leaving you vulnerable to dehydration, insomnia, sluggish digestion, disorientation, and jet lag.

Here are some tips to tackle jet lag while travelling:

- Stay hydrated and avoid caffeine and alcohol.

- Eat lightly. Put a "do not disturb" sign on your lap or table if you don't want meals.

- If you need to work, do so and then put your laptop and papers away and choose some good in-flight entertainment or listen to music or read a book. Don't doze off in front of a film. If you are tired, switch the film off and prepare to rest.

- Get up and move regularly.

- Use aromatherapy oils (lavender to help you rest or eucalyptus to ease your breathing).

- Try a deep roots meditation when taking off and landing. Close your eyes and breathe deeply. Focus on the natural rhythm of your breathing. As you breathe out, imagine putting down roots that reach all the way to the centre of the Earth, anchoring you to its core.

- Use an eye mask and ear plugs.

And here are some tips for when you arrive:

- Hold off on napping until it is time to sleep. Synchronize to the time zone of your destination.

- Eat lightly and hydrate yourself.

- Move as much as possible, preferably outdoors in nature.

- Avoid taking any medication to help you sleep. Put the emphasis on *resting* rather than sleeping.

Conclusion

Something rather magical happened during the writing of this book; I have never slept so deeply. I awoke every night and listened to birds singing – usually around 3am – before sliding effortlessly back into velvety sleep. I love waking in the early hours because I know my return to sleep will be easy and I just want to savour those few delicious seconds before I sink down again.

Jealous? Don't be. It hasn't always been this way. I was once told, "You'll always have sleep problems. It seems to run in your family." What also ran in my family was a deep lack of rootedness and safety, and that was where the real work lay. My journey of healing took decades and it finally brought me the *sattvic* sleep that I needed and craved. Your journey doesn't need to take that long. I have learned so much and it is my immense privilege to share these things with you.

Our sleep has become so unnatural and medicalized. It's time to change that.

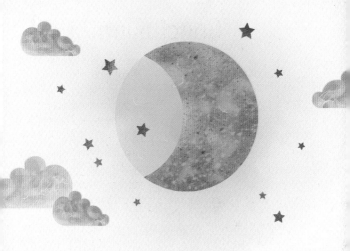

I believe our body has everything that it needs to sleep deeply, we just need to know how to trigger it. My best intention is that this little book will help you to have the natural sleep that you deserve by showing you how to activate this innate ability. It lies within you…and it's time to reclaim it.

With deep blessings,

Nerina Ramlakhan

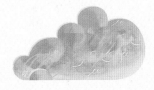

Acknowledgements

Some very special people helped me to keep my roots deep while writing, and for that I am eternally grateful. My wise and beautiful daughter Maya, who continually reminds me that "You can't give birth without some pain, mum!". My soul sisters Carolyn Kolasinski and Gosia Gorna for their unwavering belief. Lisa Lewisohn for her steadiness in holding the fort and protecting the diary so I can write. My agent Valeria Huerta, who was there just at the right time. Huge thanks to my editor Leanne Bryan who sought me out and supported my vision wholeheartedly and Polly Poulter and the team who made it come together seamlessly – you've all been brilliant to work with.

Thanks to all the mothers whose love and energy has guided me throughout this journey of surrender into *sattvic* sleep. Anandamayi Ma, who arrived just at the right moment; Lakshmi Ma and Saraswati Ma, who smile at me always; Durga Ma, who never lets me give up; my late sister Nirvana, whose maternal energy is with me always; and my own beloved mother, whose spirit only grows stronger.